COOKBOOK FOR BEGINNERS ON THE MEDIEVAL DIET

Mary M. Ratliff

Contents

Chapter One

INTRODUCTION

The Mediterranean diet is more of a lifestyle than a food "rules" diet. Its purpose is to promote the nutritious foods that people eat in the traditional areas around the Mediterranean Sea. It contains a variety of whole grains, fruits, vegetables, beans, and lentils, as well as healthy fats such as olive oil and nuts. It has a reasonable quantity of chicken, turkey, eggs, and fermented dairy, such as yoghurt or kefir, while avoiding red meat, sweets, and processed foods. Furthermore, the diet stresses the importance of cooking at home, eating with others, and getting regular exercise, such as walking.

The Mediterranean diet is rich in flavorful foods such as fruits, vegetables, whole grains, and heart-healthy fats.

It's also linked to a slew of advantages, including the ability to boost brain function, promote heart health, and regulate blood sugar levels.

2   COOKBOOK FOR BEGINNERS ON THE MEDIEVAL DIET

Despite the fact that there are no set rules for how to follow the Mediterranean diet, there are many general guidelines you may follow to incorporate the diet's principles into your everyday routine.

This book takes a closer look at the Mediterranean diet, how to follow it, and how it might affect your health, primarily for beginners and expert users.

WHERE DOES THE MEDITERRANEAN DIET COME FROM?

The Mediterranean diet is based on traditional foods that people ate in countries that border the Mediterranean Sea, such as France, Spain, Greece, and Italy.

The folks were exceptonally healthy, according to the researchers, with a minimal risk of several chronic diseases.

The diet usually encourages fruits, vegetables, whole grains, legumes, nuts, seeds, and heart-healthy fats, despite the fact that there are no strict rules or standards. Food that has been processed, added sugar, or refined grains should be avoided.

Numerous studies have now shown that eating a Mediterranean diet may help people lose weight and prevent heart attacks, strokes, type 2 diabetes, and premature death.

For this reason, the Mediterranean diet is often suggested for those seeking to improve their health and protect themselves against cardiovascular disease.

Benefits that may be generally accur

A long list of health advantages has been connected to the Mediterranean diet.

health hear

The Mediterranean diet has been extensively investigated for its capacity to boost cardiovascular health.

In fact, evidence suggests that the Mediterranean diet may be associated with a reduced risk of heart disease and stroke.

One research compared the effects of the Mediterranean diet versus a low-fat diet, finding that the Mediterranean diet was more successful in slowing plaque buildup in the arteries, which is a key risk factor for heart disease.

Other studies show that the Mediterranean diet may help lower datolec and ytolec blood pressure, which is good for heart health.

Suppports healthy blood level

The Mediterranean diet promotes a wide variety of nutrient-dense foods, such as fruits, vegetables, nuts, seeds, whole grains, and heart-healthy fats.

As a result, following the eating pattern may help table blood ugar level and prevent type 2 diabetes.

Several studies have shown that the Mediterranean diet may lower fasting blood sugar levels and improve hemoglobin A1C levels, a marker used to track long-term blood sugar control.

The Mediterranean diet has also been shown to reduce insulin resistance, a condition that impairs the body's ability to regulate blood sugar levels effectively via null hormones.

Protect your brain's performance.

Several studies suggest that the Mediterranean diet is good for brain health and may even guard against cognitive loss as you age.

For example, a research including 512 people found that better adherence to the Mediterranean diet was linked to greater memory and lower levels of many risk factors for Alzheimer's disease.

Other studies have linked the Mediterranean diet to lower levels of dementia, cognitive impairment, and Alzheimer's disease.

Furthermore, one large research found that adhering to the Mediterranean diet was associated with improvements in cognitive function, memory, attention, and processing speed in healthy older adults.

The Medterranean SHOPPING GUIDE Det LÉT It assists you in sticking to your plan, saving money, and reducing the temptation to throw less-healthy food in our cart due to a promotion. You've most likely heard that it's healthier to shop around the perimeter of the grocery store. While it's true that fresh produce, seafood, eggs, dairy, and meat are found in the outside edges, the inner aisles also have plenty of good options! Canned and dried beans, frozen fruits and vegetables, whole grains such as oatmeal and quinoa, nut and nut butter, olive oil, olives, and canned seafood may all be found in the middle aisles. To stay on track, avoid going to the store hungry, shop with a plan, and just travel down the essential aisles to get the food on your plate to avoid unnecessary (and sometimes unhealthy) items. Exact items that belong to the Mediterranean diet are controversial, mainly due to country differences.

Most studies found that those who ate a diet high in healthy plant foods and low in animal products and meat were healthier. Eating fish and sea food at least twice a week is recommended.

The Medterranean lifetyle also entails regular physical exercise, sharing meals with others, and reducing stress levels.

You may mix fresh, frozen, dried, and canned fruits and vegetables, but read the package labels for added sugar and salt.

Your diet should ideally consist of the following healthy Mediterranean foods:

Protein

Liberally

On occassion, Bean Lentl Chckpea Tofu Tempeh Setan Seafood CHICKEN FH Rarely, if ever, red meat (beef and pork) Bacon is a term that refers to a variety of meat products that have been processed (e.g., chicken nuggets)

The words "old" and "fat" are two words that come to mind while thinking about food.

Extra-vrgn olve ol Avocado and avocado olve

Margarne Butter with Tran fat

VegetableS and FRUIT

Liberally

Zucchini, eggplant, bell peppers, artichokes, and dark greens are examples of non-traditional vegetables.

Starchy vegetableS, such as weet potatoes, potatoes, and root vegetableS

Fruit, such as peaches, cherries, apricots, and berries (such as strawberries, raspberries, blueberries, and blackberries)

Occasionally

Rarely or never, there are no off-lmt fruits or vegetables.

Nothing is off-limits when it comes to fruits and vegetables!

Nuts and Seeds are two types of nuts and seeds that may be found in nature.

Liberally

Chapter Two

TABOULI SALAD

Bread made from whole grains (look for whole wheat flour as the first ingredient) Farro, bulgur wheat, barley, and unoa are examples of whole grains.

Breakfast (choose between steel-cut or traditional) Occasionally Pata (where possible, prefer whole-wheat pata) Couscous

Polenta cracker worldworldworldworldworldworldworldworldworldwor

cereal all-bran Waffle and pancakes are seldom, if ever, free. cereals that have been ugar-weetened cracker and other nack food

Dairy

Liberally

These are also ingested in the form of moderation.

Plain Greek yogurt may be found on occasion.

Plan rcotta and cottage cheee Mlk Brie, feta, or goat cheese (along with any other cheeses you like) Ice cream Sweetened yoghurt Processed cheese (such as American) Rarely or never

Sweeteners

Liberally

In moderation, they are consumed. Occasionally\sHoney

Rarely or Never White ugar Condment and Sauces A tiny quantity of added ugar, for example, in coffee or tea

Liberally

Tomato auce (no extra virgin olive oil) Balsamic vinegar with pesto

sauce barbecue

Teryak sauce for ktchup

Drinks

Liberally

coffee water Tea\sOccasionally

alcohol red wne or any alcohol Fruit juice is seldom, if ever, consumed.

weetened coffee bottled

Spce (herbs)

Liberally

pce and all dry herb Garlic, herbs, and herbs Occasionally

tate salt ingredients

Never or RARELY

There's no need to keep them out of your diet.

Day Mediterranean Diet Eating Plan Below is an example menu for two weeks of meals on the Mediterranean diet.

Feel free to adjust the quantity and food choices to suit your needs and tastes, and add nack as necessary.

1st day Snack: coffee or tea with a bowl of oatmeal topped with berres Almonds or walnuts, by the handful

Lunch Half a turkey and a cup of lentil soup Snack hummus-dipped sliced carrots, bell peppers, and cucumbers

Tew dnner vege and wean

Day 2 – Breakfast or tea with plain Greek yogurt and walnuts drizzled on top Snack Lunch of roasted chicken Yeterday's vegetable and bean tew

Chapter Three

MEDITERRANEAN BREAKFAST EGGS

Snip a peach (or an apple, depending on the occasion)

Dinner Roasted chicken with pita bread, tzatziki sauce (a yogurt-based sauce), and a side salad

3rd day Smoothie made with your favorite milk, fruits, and nuts

On top of whole-grain crackers, snack 14 avocados mashed with lime juice and salt. Snack: Lunch Three-Bean Stack topped with a dollop of pistachio and served on a whole-grain bun olve and free vegetable package

Salmon for Dinner with Farro and Roasted Zucchini and Eggplant

Breakfast on Day 4 trawberre, Lunch with Snack Pistachios Salad with feta, roasted red peppers, un-dried tomatoes, and olive oil, lentl-baed Snack yogurt made with fresh fruit and greek yogurt

Grilled prawns with sautéed kale and polenta for dinner.

Breakfast day 5 A morning bowl of leftover farro (from dinner on day 3) topped with a poached egg and a few slices of avocado Snack walnuts with dried apricot

Qunoa, bean, and vegetable salad served with a whole-grain piece of bread Whole-gran crackers snacks with black bean dip

Dinner Marinated, grilled chicken knuckles served with bulgur wheat and a cucumber and red onion salad

6th day Breakfast Coffee or tea wth moked salmon, capers, and tomato slices

Snack Fruit grown in the field (such as a peach or two apricots in the summer; a pear in the winter) Lunch Medterranean bean alad and whole-grain crackers

Olives with a snack piece of cheese

Moroccan lamb tew wth couscous dnner

7th day of the week Coffee or tea with Greek yogurt, sunflower seeds, and raspberries Snack Pistachios and sloughed orange

Lunch A whole-grain bread with chopped tomatoes, cheese, and olives Snack Luupn bean Dinner, packaged and flavored vegetable tew and red lentl

Breakfast on the 8th day 2 eggs with sautéed greens (pnach or kale) and an orange Snack chcckpea roast

Snack: Lunch Leftover lamb tew from day 6 supper dark chocolate mixed nut

Dinner Zucchini, roasted potatoes, and baked white fish

Day 9 Snack Mini peppers stuffed with hummus Breakfast Smoothe prepared with your choice of milk, frozen cookies, banana, and cocoa powder

Tuna salad with olive oil, dred herb, olives, and un-dred tomatoes served over a bed of pnach with assorted vegetables and whole grain crackers

Snack a sliver of cheese paired with a sliver of fruit

Dnner Tuscan white bean soup with whole grain bread

Breakfast day 10 coffee or tea and a bowl of oatmeal topped with ran and cruhed walnuts, with a drizzle of honey if desired

Snack Lunch Leftover Tuscan whete bean oup from denner on day 9 with greek yogurt and a piece of fruit

Snack Hummu with Iced raw vegetables like red peppers, celery, and cucumber Dinner Garlc lemon chicken thighs with arugula and Irael cooucou

Breakfast on Day 11 Coffee or tea wth avocado and a slice of vege freshtata Snack Use nut butter as a topping.

Lunch Prepared dolma with hummu and pita (search for these packed lettuce leaves in the prepared food section at certain supermarkets).

Snack Iced vegger greek yogurt dp

Dinner Seafood stew (shrimp and mussels in a tomato sauce)

Breakfast day 12 A small dish of ricotta topped with fruit (berries, pears, or fresh apricot) and a cup of coffee or tea and honey drizzle

Snack hazelnut, ptacho, almond, or a mix)

Lunch GreeK pata alad (whole-grain pasta with red onion, tomato, Kalamata olives, and feta) served on a bed of Romaine Snack Fruit Salad

Dinner: eafood stew left over from the previous day's dinner

Day 13: Coffee with Breakfast Snack: tea and oatmeal wth nut butter and blueberries Greek yogurt container

Lunch Salad salmon and a cup of bean-based soup Snack On whole-grain crackers, smashed avocado Shakshuka for Dinner (baked egg with tomato sauce) erved over polenta, topped wth feta

Breakfast on 14th day toasted whole-grain bread with ricotta and licked fruit. Snack maxed nuts and drewn cranberries

Lunch Quinoa bowl with roasted sweet potatoes, goat cheese, and walnuts Snack Olve and a few hummu pta chips

Artichoke and cannellini bean spaghetti with breadcrumbs and Parmesan

tip for medterranean creatng Plan Det

The good news is that, since it's a way of eating rather than a set of rules, you may totally customize it to your preferences. There's no going off the wagon and feeling like a failure if you don't follow this to a T. According to Berman, it is a diet that will last you a lifetime. Still, here are five crucial pointers to help you get started: Eat more legumes.

They're not just a snack that you're probably not getting enough of anyway, but they're also "budget friendly and pack a great nutritional punch," according to Berman, who adds that they're high in fiber and protein and low in fat. Lentils, dried peas, beans, and chickpeas (such as hummu) are among them.

Don't go overboard with the booze.

One common medterranean det misconception is that those who follow it drink a lot of red wine. "Alcohol is an integral component of our way of life. If you drink wine, limit yourself to a moderate amount while eating and enjoying a meal with friends or family," advises Berman.

Make a decision with meat.

According to Paravante-Hargtt, traditionally, people only eat meat for special occasions, such as a Sunday dinner, and even then only in small amounts. Incorporate more plant-based meats into your day (think: beaan, tofu, or seitan). "Going vegan one day a week is a good place to start," he says. If you must eat meat, choose skinless chicken and save red meat for once or twice a month.

Reduce the amount of sugary foods you consume.

Make desserts a special occasion meal, just as you would meat. That doesn't mean you can't have a little sugar in your coffee if you want, but Paravante-Hargtt says, "but on a daily basis, there isn't much sugar eaten."

Preheat the oven to 350 degrees Fahrenheit and bake with olive oil.

Extra-vrgn olve all the olve you cook wth While doing it with the ol can lead to weight gain (it's a fat, after all, so the calories can quickly add up), it's rich in heart-healthy polyunsaturated and monounsaturated fat, so you can feel good about keeping a little harm. You can also use it in cold applications to make ice cream or to drzzl cooked vegetables or dhee.

Breakfast & Breakfast Drnk MEDITERRANEAN DIET RECIPES

INGREDIENTS: ay heet pan baked egg and vege

1 green bell pepper, peeled and finely chopped 1 red bell pepper, cored and thinly sliced 1 medium red onion, halved and thinly sliced 2 teaspoon za'atar blend, 1 teaspoon ground cumin, and 1 teaspoon Aleppo chili pepper

Early Harvet Greek extra virgin olive oil (I used Early Harvet Greek extra vrgn olve ol 6 oz.

a large handful of freshly chopped parley 1 Roma tomato, diced Crumbled feta, a pinch of salt and pepper to taste (optional) INSTRUCTIONS

Preheat oven to 400 degrees Fahrenheit (200 degrees Celsius).

In a large mixing bowl, combine Iced bell peppers (all colors). Onions that have been red should be added. 1 teaspoon za'atar, 1 teaspoon cumin, and 1 teaspoon Aleppo chili pepper (reserve the remaining za'atar for later). DRIZZLE WITH EXTRA VIGOROUS OLIVE OIL. To coat, to coat, to coat, to coat, to coat, to coat, to coat, to coat

Fill a large heat pan halfway with pepper and onion medley. One layer should be spread out. For 10 to 15 minutes in a preheated oven.

Remove the pan from the oven and set it aside for a moment. Make 6 "holes" or "openings" in the roasted vegetables with care. Carefully crack each egg into a hole, keeping the yolk in tact (it helps to crack the egg in a small dish to ld carefully into each hole.)

Return the pan to the oven and bake until the egg whites are slightly firm. Wait for the yokes to turn the way you want (anywhere between 5 and 8 minutes).

remove from oven To your lark, add a few eggs. 1 teaspoon za'atar, sprinkling all over Combine the parsley, diced tomatoes, and a pinch of feta. Immediately serve!

Variations: The baked egg recpe can really be made by you. Change up the vegetables to use what you have on hand; adjust the roasting time accordingly (examples include zucchini, broccoli, yellow squash, and spring onions). You can also experiment with different flavor combinations (for example, if you enjoy smoky flavors, use smoked paprika with salt and pepper). For a Moroccan twist, try a hara spice blend with a pinch of turmerc. For a touch of Italian, use dried oregano or bal.)

Tp: TPP: This is a simple enough recipe to prepare the day before you want to serve it. It will look better then, but if you want to try and work ahead, you can prep the peppers and onions ahead of time and store them in the refrigerator overnight. You can roast the vegetables the night before or the day before. In a light-ld container, store them in the fridge. When ready, spread on a hot pan and prepare as directed in Step 5. Because you'll have to clean the sheet pan twice, it's not a good idea.

Storage Tips: Leftovers can be stored in the refrigerator for up to three days. To tore, divide the leftovers into gla contaner with light lds, however many meals you plan on eating, and refrigerate. At room temperature or slightly warmed, this dish is delectable. Use a kllet on medium heat for a few minutes to warm up.

INGREDIENTS FOR EASY HUMMU RecP

3 cups peeled cooked chickpeas (from 1 to 14 cup dry chickpeas or high-quality canned chickpeas) For more information on how to cook and peel chicken, see the recipe notes.)

1–2 garlic cloves, minced 3–4 ice cubes 1 cup (79 g) tahn paste

12 tsp koher alt Juce of 1 lemon Hot water

Sumac INSTRUCTIONS EARLY Harvet Greek extra virgin olive oil

In a food processor's bowl, combine chickpeas and minced garlic. Puree until you have a smooth, pudding-like consistency.

Add the cubes, tahini, salt, and lemon juice while the processor is running. Blend for approximately 4 minutes. Check, and if the consistency is still too high, repeat the process with a small amount of hot water added gradually. Blend until you get the silky smooth consistency you desire.

Add a generous drizzle of Early Harvet EVOO and spread in a serving bowl. If you want, you can add a few chickpeas to the mix. On top, sprinkling umac. Warm pita wedges and your favorite vegetables are a delicious combination.

INGREDIENTS FOR

1 mall red bell pepper, chopped (about 34 cup) 12 cherry tomatoes, halved 1 hallot, fnely chopped 6 to 10 ptted kala-mata olve, chopped parley LEAVES, FRESHLY CRUMBLED To your 8 large eggs, add a handful of crumbled feta. 12 tsp salt and pepper 14 tp ground turmerc (optional) Spanh paprka

INSTRUCTIONS

Preheat your oven to 350 degrees F and place a rack in the middle.

Make a 12-cup muffin pan (or 12 individual muffin cups) similar to this one. Extra virgin olive oil should be used as a brush.

Distribute the peppers, tomatoes, halloumi, olives, chicken (or turkey), parsley, and crumbled feta among the 12 cups (they should fill up to about? of the way).

Add eggs, salt, pepper, and spices to a large measuring cup or a mixing bowl. To combine, work hard.

Pour the egg mixture over each cup gently, leaving a little amount of space at the top (approximately 34% of the way or more).

To assist catch any pll, place a muffin pan or muffin cup on top of a heet pan. Bake for 25 minutes, or until the egg muffins are set, in a preheated oven.

Allow a few minutes to cool before loosening the edges of each muffin with a small butter knife. erve and remove form pan!Eat them in moderation, even though they may be a part of every day.

Occasionally

Almonds\s

Pistachios Hazelnuts Walnuts

Cashews (as well as any other raw nut) Never or Rarely

Trail mx with a sweetener nut butters sweetened Nuts with a sugar coating

Grains

Liberally

Chapter Four

SHAKSHUKA

INGREDIENTS: foul mudamma (Egyptian fava bean)

2 can fava beans (each can should be 13 to 15 ounces) (see note on using dry fava beans)

12 carrot of water 1 to 2 heat pepper, chopped (jalapenos will work here) Kohr alt 12 to 1 teapoon ground 1 large lemon juice of Extra vrgn olve ol (Early Harvet) 2 garlic cloves, sliced 1 cup parsley tomato, chopped

Serving Instructions:

Warm pt bread Sliced tomatoes Cucumbers Olives INSTRUCTIONS

Place the fava beans and 12 cup water in a cast iron pan or aucepan. Warm on medum-heat. Season to taste with kosher salt and freshly ground black pepper. To mash the fava beans, use a potato maher or fork. Add the hot peppers and garlic to a mortar and pestle. Smash. To mix, add a juice of one lemon.

Over the fava bean, pour the garlc and hot pepper auce. generou drzzle extra vrgn olve Top with chopped parsley, diced tomatoes, and, if desired, a few lces of hot peppers.

Serve with pita bread, chopped vegetables, and olives as a side dish.

Two banana date-making INGREDIENTS

4 pitted frozen bananas Medjool date (you can chop them up a little if they're too big.)

14 cup tahini (I used Soom)

12 cup unsweetened almond milk 14 cup crushed ice Pnch ground cnnamon, more INSTRUCTIONS

for

In a blender, combine the thawed frozen bananas with the other ingredients. Blend until a smooth and creamy hake is obtained.

Switch the banana date hake to a serving cup and sprinkle with a touch of ground cinnamon. Enjoy!

INGREDIENTS FOR

(I used Private Reserve EVOO) Extra virgin olive oil 1 large yellow onion, chopped green peppers, chopped 2 garlic cloves, peeled and chopped 1 tablespoon ground cinnamon

1 tbsp paprika (sweet)

12 tp ground combination

(Optional) Pnch red pepper flake

6 Vine-ripe tomatoes, chopped (about 6 cups chopped tomatoes) salt and pepper

tomato auce (12 cup) 6 large eggs

14 cup freshly chopped parsley leaves (about 0.2 oz or 5 g)

14 cup freshly chopped mint leaves (about 0.2 oz or 5 g)

INSTRUCTIONS

3 to Combine the onion, green peppers, garlic, spices, pnch salt, and pepper. Cook, stirring regularly, for about 5 minutes, or until the veggies are softened.

Tomatoes and tomato sauce are added last. Cover and set aside for 15 minutes to allow the flavors to mingle. Remove the cover and continue to simmer for a few minutes more to enable the mixture to decrease and thicken. Taste the sauce and adjust the seasoning to your preference.

Make 6 indentations, or "wells," in the tomato mixture with a wooden spoon (make sure they're evenly spaced). In each indention, gently crack an egg.

Reduce the heat to low and cook the egg whites until they are set.

add the new parley and mnt. More black pepper or crushed red pepper may be used if desired. Warm pta, challah brew, or your favorite cruty brew will be served.

INGREDIENTS FOR EASY GREEN JUICE RECIPE

1 kale (about 5 oz)

1 Granny smith apple (or any large apple) 1 nch pece freh gnger, peeled 12 big English cucumber 5 celery stalks, ends trmmed 1 oz. parsley (handful)

INSTRUCTIONS

Clean the veggies by washing and rinsing them. I like chopping them up into big chunks. Add to a blender and blend on high (or add to a juicer and juice in the order listed.)

Simply pour the green juice into glasses and enjoy right away if you used a juicer. The juice will be thicker if you used a blender. You may sift it through a fine mesh sieve and then press the pulp into the sieve with the back of a spoon to extract as much liquid as possible. Pour the juice into glasses and enjoy!

Chapter Five

A M dt rr n n BRUNCH BOARD

1 falafel recepton

1 clac hummus recipe (or roasted green garbanzo hummus, roasted red pepper hummus) 1 Recpe of Baba Ganoush

1 LabneH Recpe or Feta CHEESE Recipe for 1 Taboul

1 to 2 tomatoes, cut 1 English cucumber, sliced 6 to 7 Radh, halved or sliced

Olives (I like a combination of green and kalamata olives) Muhrooms or marinated artichokes ,

Pta Bread, split into quarters Grape (palette cleaner) Early Harvest EVOO with Za'atar For garnish, fresh herb

INSTRUCTIONS

Note: Plan ahead of time to make the majority of these for a fast and simple assembly. Look up note in the dictionary.

Follow the recipe to make the falafel. Before soaking the chickpeas, you should start at least the night before. For working forward, see the notes below. (Falafel may also be purchased in a local Middle Eastern store.)

Baba ganouh according to the recpe. Both of these may be prepared the night before and stored in the refrigerator. If you want to spice things up, try roasted garlic hummus or roasted red pepper hummus. (Use high-quality store-bought hummu if you don't have time.)

Choose feta cheese or make Labneh ahead of time using this recipe.

Prepare the tabouli as directed in the recipe. Can be prepared a few days ahead of time and refrigerated in tall glass containers.

Place hummus, baba ganoush, olive oil, za'atar, and tabouli in bowls to assemble the Mediterranean breakfast board. To create a focal point, place the biggest bowl in the middle of a large wooden board or platter. Arrange the remaining bowls on various parts of the board or plate to create movement and symmetry. Fill in the gaps between the bowls with the remaining components, such as falafel, diced vegetables, and patty bread. If desired, top with grapes and fresh herbs. Salad and Side Salad

INGREDIENTS:

6 Roma tomatoes, diced (about 3 cups)

12 to 34 cup chopped fresh parsley leaves koher salt Try a robut like Greek robut with sumac tablepoon extra vrgn olve ol Hojiblanca or Early Harvest EVOO from Spain.

2 teapot lemon juice, freshly squeezed INSTRUCTIONS

Toss the chopped tomatoes, cucumbers, and parsley into a large mixing bowl. Season with kosher salt and freshly ground pepper. Set ade for 5 minutes

Combine the umac, olive oil, and lemon juice in a large mixing bowl. Give the alad a moderate squeeze. Enjoy!

dp INGREDIENTS hunky ctru avocado

2 navel oranges, peeled and diced 2 avocados, pitted, peeled, and diced 12 cup/ 60 g chopped red onions

12 clantro cup

12 cubes/7 g chopped fresh meat 12 cubes/400 g walnut hearts, chopped Salt and pepper 34 teaspoons Sumac 1 34 oz/ 49 g crumbled feta cheese INSTRUCTIONS Cayenne Juce of 1 lemon Generou drzzle Early Harvet Greek extra virgin olive oil

In one large bowl, combine oranges, avocado, red onion, fresh herbs, and walnuts. Season with salt, pepper, a pinch of cayenne, and a pinch of sugar.

Add a generous drizzle of Early Harvest EVOO and lime juice. to combine in a gently way On top, add feta cheese. Serve with your favorite healthy side dish.

INGREDIENTS FOR A FAST Oven-Roasted Tomatoes Recpe

2 lb Campar tomatoeS, halved 2–3 garlic cloves, Kosher salt and black pepper, minced

2 teaspoons fresh thyme, stems removed 1 teaspoon sumac 12 teaspoons dry chili pepper flake Crumbled feta cheese, optional INSTRUCTIONS: Extra virgin olive oil, I used Private Reerve Greek extra virgin olive oil

Preheat the oven to 450 degrees Fahrenheit (230 degrees Celsius).

In a large mixing bowl, place the tomato halves. mnced garlc, alt, pepper, fresh thyme, and pce Drizzle ualty additional vrgn olve in a big amount, around 14 cup or more. Toss to evenly distribute the ingredients.

Place the potatoes on a rimmed baking sheet. Spread the tomatoes in a single layer with the flesh side up.

Cook for 30 to 35 minutes in a preheated oven, or until the tomatoes have collapsed to your desired consistency.

remove yourself from the heat If you're going to serve it right away, add some more fresh thyme and a few sprinkling of feta cheese. Warm or room temperature is OK.

INGREDIENTS FOR THE TRADITIONAL GREEK SALAD

1 medium red onon 4 Medium jucy tomatoes 1 English cucumber (hot houe cucumber) trped pattern partially peeled 1 cored green bell pepper

4 tablepoon ualty extra virgin olve ol I ued Early Harvest Greek olve ol 1-2 tablepoon red wine venegar 1-2 tablepoon red wine venegar

Do not shred the Greek cheese blocks; instead, leave them in large pieces with 12 tablespoons oregano. INSTRUCTIONS

Half the red onion and then slice it into half-moon slices. (To remove the edge, place the sliced onion in a oluton of iced water and set aside for a few minutes before adding to the salad.)

Cut the tomatoes into wedges or large pieces (I rounded some and wedged the rest).

Half-lengthwise cut the partly peeled cucumber, then slice into thick halves (at least 12" thick).

The pepper nto ringing bell is thinly Iced.

Everything should be placed in a large salad dish. Add a large handful of kalamata olives that have been ptted. Season with a touch of kosher salt and a dash of dried oregano.

Pour the olive oil and red wine vinegar over the whole salad. Give everything a little toss to combine (do not overmix; the alad isn't supposed to be touched much).

Add a few more dreed oregano blocks on top of the feta blocks. With crusty bread, if desired.

INGREDIENTS

8 oz. baby bella mushrooms, cleaned and trimmed 12 oz. baby potatoes, cubed (Or cut potatoes in half or cubes depending on size). You want them to be tinier.)

a 12-ounce bottle Campar tomatoeS, grape tomatoeS, and cherry tomatoeS 2 zucchini or ummer uah, peeled and cut into 1-inch pieces 10-12 large garlic cloves

Extra vrgn olve ol

12 tblsp oregano (dried) 1 tsp thyme (dried) Frehly grated salt and ppepper Parmean cheese for optonal development Alternative: crushed red pepper flake

INSTRUCTIONS

Preheat the oven to 425 degrees Fahrenheit (230 degrees Celsius).

In a large mixing basin, combine the mushrooms, veggies, and cheese. Drizzle olive oil generally (about 14 cup olive oil). Add the oregano, thyme, salt, and pepper once it has been drained.
ttttttttttttttttttttttt

Only put the potatoes on a lightly greased baking pan. Cook for 10 minutes in a preheated oven. Remove the muhroom and the remaining vegetables from the heat. Return to the oven and continue to roast for another 20 minutes or until the vegetables are fork-tender (some charring is OK!)

Serve immediately with a sprinkling of grated Parmesan cheese and roasted red pepper flakes (optional).

INGREDIENTS FOR A Which Bean Salad

2 cannellini beans, drained and rinsed well 1 English cucumber, diced 10 ounces grape or cherry tomatoes, chopped 4 green onions, chopped 1 cup chopped fresh parsley 15 to 20 mint leaves, chopped 1 teaspoon Za'atar, 12 teaspoons Sumac, and 12 teaspoons Aleppo For other choices, see the notes.)

Extra vrgn olve ol (I used Early Harvest EVOO) OPTIONAL INSTRUCTIONS FOR Feta CHEESE

In a large mixing bowl, combine the white beans, cucumbers, tomatoes, green onion, parsley, and mnt. Lemon zet should be added to the mix. Season with salt and pepper, then add the za'atar, umac, and Aleppo pepper.

Finish with a generous drizzle of extra virgin olive oil (2 to 3 tablespoons) and a squeeze of lemon juice.

Give the alad a good stir. Taste and adjust your eaoning. If desired, add feta cheese. (Let the salad sit for 30 minutes or so before serving for the finest taste.) (For further information, see note.)

NOTES

Tip from the kitchen This salad will taste better if you leave it for 30 minutes or so to allow the flavors to blend. Make it 1 night ahead of time, cover it, and keep it refrigerated until ready to use. When I'm ready to serve, I usually keep the feta and mix it in.

Spice Variations: You may alter the proportions in the recipe to suit your preferences. Also fantastic choices are oregano and cumin. Add a pinch of crushed red pepper flakes if you want a little more heat.

To make dry beans, follow these instructions: To get started, you'll need about 1 cup dry beans. Overnight, soak the bread in plenty of water. Keep them in the refrigerator to thaw. Drining is required prior to cooking. After draining the beans, put them in a large enough pot to expand. Bring to a boil with a cover of about 2 inches of cold water. Reduce the heat, cover, and cook, stirring occasionally, for 1 to 12 hours, or until the beans are tender. Allow the beans to cool slightly before using in the salad, and discard any excess water. Follow the directions on the alad recpe.

INGREDIENTS: Roasted cauliflower and chickpea stew

12 tp turmerc (ground) 12 tblsp cumin powder 12 tblsp cinnamon powder 1 tsp sweet paprika 1 tsp ground corander

1 tblsp. cayenne pepper (optional)

12 tblsp. cardamom powder

1 whole head cauflower, divided into small florets, medium-sized bulk carrots, peeled and cut into 12" pieces pepper and salt

Private olve extra vrgn 2 14-ounce cans chickpeas, drained and rinsed 1 large wet onion, chopped garlic cloves, chopped 1 tomatoe juced 28-oz can

12 CUPS parsley leaves, tem REMOVED, ROUGHLY CRUMBLED Optional: toated lvered almounds

Optional: toasted pine nut INSTRUCTIONS

Preheat the oven to 475 degrees Fahrenheit (230 degrees Celsius).

Toss together the spices in a small bowl.

Arrange the cauliflower flowers and carrot pieces on a large, lightly oiled baking sheet. SEASONING WITH SALT AND PEPPER Add a smidgeon more than 12 teaspoons of the spice mix. Drizzle a generous amount of olive oil over the cauflower and carrots, then toss to coat evenly.

Cook for 20 minutes in a 475°F heated oven, or until the carrots and cauliflower are softened and color has developed. Take the pan off the heat and set it aside for the time being. Switch off the oven.

2 tablepoon olive oil, heated in a large cat ron pot or a Dutch oven Add the onions and cook for 3 minutes before adding the garlc and remaining pce. Cook for another 2-3 minutes on medium-high, constantly stirring.

Add the chckpea and canned tomatoe now. alt and pepper seasonings Roasted cauliflower and carrots should be stirred in. Bring to a boil, then reduce to medium-low heat, cover, and cook for an additional 20 minutes. Check the stew occasionally, stir it in, and add a splash of water if necessary. Remove the food from the heat and place it in a serving bowl. Garnh wth free parley and toated nut (optional.) Serve hot with a side of warm pita bread or over some quick-cooked cooucous.

INGREDIENTS FOR

4 fresh Roma tomatoes, very finely chopped 1/2 cup extra fine bulgur

very finely chopped bunche parley, part of the tem removed, washed, and well-dried, very finely chopped 12-15 fresh mint leaves, tem removed, washed, and well-dried, very finely chopped 4 green

3-4 tablespoons lime juice (lemon juice, if desired) Extra virgin olive oil, early harvest SERVING INSTRUCTIONS FOR Romane Lavage LEAVES

Soak the bulgur wheat in water for 5-7 minutes after washing. Drink thoroughly (use your hand to squeeze out any excess water from the bulgur). Remove yourself from the picture.

As stated above, chop the vegetables, herbs, and green onions very finely. To drain excess juice, place the tomatoes in a colander.

In a mixing bowl or dish, combine the chopped vegetables, dill, and green onions. Toss in the bulgur and season with salt and pepper. gently mx

Mix in the lime juice and olive oil until thoroughly combined.

Cover the tart and refrigerate for 30 minutes for the best results. Transfer to a platter for ervent. Serve the tabouli with a side of pta and romaine lettuce leaves, which act as a wrap or "boat" for the tabouli if desired.

Other appetizers to serve alongside the tartare: Hummu, Baba Ganoush, or Roasted Red Pepper Hummu

INGREDIENTS IN A Medterranean Watemelon ALAD

Vnagrette for Honey

honey, 2 tblsp

2 tbsp lime juice 1 to 2 tablespoons extra virgin olive oil (I used Greek Early Harvest) pinch of salt

12 watermelon, peeled and cubed 1 English (or Hot House) cucumber, cubed (approximately 2 cupfuls) 15 fresh mint leaves, 15 fresh basil leaves, 12 cup crumbled feta cheese, additional to your liking INSTRUCTIONS

Whisk the honey, lime juice, olive oil, and a pinch of salt together in a small bowl. For a moment, set ade.

Combine the watermelon, cucumbers, and fresh herbs in a large bowl or on a serving platter with de.

Drizzle the honey vinaigrette over the watermelon salad and toss gently to combine. Serve topped with feta cheese.

INGREDIENTS: BAKED ZUCCHINI WITH PARMESAN AND THYME

3–4 zucchini, trimmed and cut lengthwise into an uarter (tck) For the Parmesan-Thyme topping, I used Private Reserve Greek extra virgin olive oil.

2 teaspoon fresh thyme leaves (no stems) 12 cup grated Parmesan 12 teaspoon weet paprika 1 teaspoon dried oregano This natural paprka was what I used. 12 teaspoon kosher black pepper

Preheat the oven to 350°F.

Combine the grated Parmesan, thyme, and spices in a mixing bowl and stir to combine.

Prepare a large baking sheet with a wire baking rack, similar to this one. Using extra virgin olive oil (or a healthy cooking spray), lightly brush the baking rack. Arrange the zucchini sticks on the baking rack, kn-de down, and bruh each zucchini stick with extra vrgn olve

Sprnkle the Parmean-thyme toppng on each zucchn stick.

Bake 15 to 20 minutes or until tender in a preheated oven. Then, for a golden crisp topping, broil for an additional 2 to 3 minutes, carefully watching.

Serve right away as an appetizer with a dipping sauce of tzatziki or hummus! Serve as a side dish alongside your preferred entree.

RECIPE INGREDIENTS BABA GANOUSH

14 cup tahini paste 2 Italian eggplants or small globe eggs I took advantage of 1 teaspoon sumac 34 teaspoon tahini 1 lemon, juice of 1 garlic clove, minced 1 tablespoon plain Greek yogurt, optional Kosher salt and black pepper Extra vrgn olve ol Toasted pine nuts for garnh, optional INSTRUCTIONS Aleppo pepper or red pepper flakes, optional

To begin, smoke or grill the eggs. Set medum-hgh on one gas burner. Place the eggplant in the appropriate location.

directly around the flame. Turn the eggplant every 5 minutes or so with a pair of tongs until it tenders and the skin is crisp on both sides (20 minutes). The eggplant should deflate and become more tethered, contrary to popular belief. You can use a grill if you don't have a gas burner. You may roast the eggplant in the oven as well (see notes).

Remove the eggplant from the heat and place it in a large condenser over a bowl to cool. Allow it cool for a few minutes before draining (it helps if you open the eggplant a bit and press on it with a knife or a spoon to assist it release its juice).

Peel the charred crusty skin off the eggplant after it is cool enough to touch (it should come off easily). Keep the kn and the tem (don't worry if a few bits of the kn remain; it only adds taste).

Into a bowl, transfer the cooked and well drained eggplant. Break it up with a fork. Toss in the tahini paste, greek yogurt (if using), salt, pepper, umac, Aleppo pepper, or crushed red pepper flakes. Using a wooden spoon or a fork, gently mix until everything is fully incorporated.

Cover the baby ganouh and chill for 30 minutes to an hour.

Transfer the baba ganouh to an rmmed ervng dh or a bowl to serve. If you want, finish with a drizzle of extra virgin olive oil and toasted pine nuts. Serve with pta wedges or pta chops and your favorite vegetables.

INGREDIENTS FOR Medterranean CHECKPEA ALAD

1 big eggplant, thinly laced (no more than 14 nches in thickness)

1 cup cooked or canned chickpeas, drained 3 tbp Za'atar spice, divided 12 English cucumber, diced 1 small red onion, split in 12 moons 1 cup chopped parsley 1 cup chopped dill

For the Garlic Vinaigrette, combine all ingredients in a mixing bowl and whisk together until smooth.

1 large lemon, juice of 1 cup Early 1-2 garlic cloves, minced EXTRA VIRGIN OLIVE OIL SALT+PEPPER INSTRUCTIONS Harvet EXTRA VIRGIN OLIVE OIL

Eggplant should be cooked (optional) Place the Iced eggplant on a big tray and prnkle generally with alt. Allow for 30 minutes to settle (the bitterness of the eggplant will "weat out" as it rests). Place a paper bag topped with paper towel on another large tray or baking sheet near the stove.

Optional: Cook Eggplant Allow time for the egg to dry. 4 to 5 ry the eggs in batches (carefully, so the kllet does not overcrowd). Turn the eggplant slices over and fry the other side when one side has become golden brown. Using a slotted patula, remove the eggplant lace and place it on the paper towel-lined tray to drain and cool.

Place the eggplant on a serving dish once it has cooled. 1 tablepoon Za'atar, sprinkling

To make chickpea salad, combine all of the ingredients in a large mixing bowl. Toss the tomatoes, cucumbers, chickpeas, red onion, parsley, and dill together in a medium mixing bowl. Mix gently with the remaining Za'atar.

Make the preparations for the dreng. Whisk together the ingredients in a small bowl. Drizzle 2 tablespoons salad dressing over the fried eggplant; pour the remaining dressing over the crisppea salad and toss to combine.

Serve the eggplant with the chickpea salad.

INGREDIENTS rpy homemade fish tck recpe rpy

1 12 lb firm fish fillet, such as almon (you may use a firm white fish fillet like cod)

1 tblsp. black pepper 1 tblsp. dreed oregano

1 tblsp. wet paprka

12 cup flour (all-purpose flour, whole wheat flour, or gluten-free flour) 1 egg, beated in 1 tablepoon water (egg wah)

12 CUP BAKED BREAD CRUMBS 12 CUP PARMESAN CHEESE

Extra virgin olive oil (I used Private Reserve Greek Extra Virgin Olive Oil) 1 lemon zette and 12 lemon juce

parley for gentlement

Servants:

INSTRUCTIONS FOR Tahn sauce or Tzatzk sauce

Preheat the oven to 450 degrees Fahrenheit (230 degrees Celsius).

Place fh flet dry on both sides and season with koher alt. Cut the fifth fillet into pieces or sticks (1 to 12 inch thick and about 3-inch long).

Combine the black pepper, oregano, and paprika in a small bowl. Fh tck on both de wth the spice mxture

Create a taton for dredging. In a small dish, sift flour. Place the egg whites in a separate dish or bowl next to the flour. Combine the breadcrumbs, parmesan cheese, and lemon zest in a separate dish. Put the egg wash next to the dish.

Coat the fh right now. To coat both sides, take a fh tck and dip it in flour; hake exce flour off. Then dip the fh stick in the egg wash, followed by the bread crumb and Parmesan mixture. To aid the coating's adhesion to the fish stick, preheat the oven to 350°F. Rep until all of the fish are covered.

Arrange a tack of coated fish on a greased baking sheet. Bruh the tops of the fish sticks with a little extra virgin olive oil (you'll want to bacally dab the salmon fish sticks with the oil so you don't wind up removing the coating).

Place the baking sheet on the oven's middle rack. Preheat the oven to 350°F and bake for 12–15 minutes. If the fish still need more color, place them under the broler very lightly (and carefully) until the fish tck develop a wonderful golden brown color.

Finish with fresh lemon juice and lemon zest. parley garnh

Serve with your favorite dipping sauce. I didn't use any sauce, but tzatziki would be delicious. Add a big salad and you've got yourself a meal (which I really like). With this almoon fh tck, make a Mediterranean white bean salad or a Greek salad.

Chicken Shawarma INGREDIENTS: Sandwiches, Soups, and Stews

34 tblsp ground cumin 34 tblsp turmerc powder 34 tblsp ground coriander 34 tblsp garlic powder 34 tblsp paprka

12 tblsp cloves (ground)

12 teaspoon cayenne pepper, or more if desired Salt

8 boneless, skinless chicken breasts 1 large onion, thinly sliced 1 large lemon, juice of the lemon extra vrgn olive oil should be saved.

SERVE

6 pta pta pta pta pta

Tahn auce or Greek au (optional) Pckle or kalmata olve

INSTRUCTIONS

Combine the corn, turmeric, cinnamon, curry powder, garbanzo bean powder, sweet paprika, and cloves in a small bowl. Set the hawarma pce mx aside for the time being.

Dry and season the chicken thighs on both sides with salt, then thinly slice into little bite-size pieces.

In a large bowl, place the chicken. To Combine the onions, lime juice, and olive oil in a large mixing bowl. To get everythng together another type of type of type of type of type Cover and chill for 3 hours or overnight (you may decrease or omit the marinating time if you don't have time).

Preheat the oven to 425 degrees Fahrenheit when you're ready. Remove the chicken from the refrigerator and let it aside for a few minutes at room temperature. On a large lightly-oiled baking sheet pan, spread the marinated chicken with the onion in one layer. Preheat the oven to 425 degrees F and roast for 30 minutes. Move the pan to the top rack and brol very brefly (watch carefully) for a more browned, crispier chicken. Remove the oven from the situation.

Preparing the pita pockets while the chicken is roasting Make tahn auce or Tztazk auce according to this recipe. Follow this recipe to make a 3-ingredient Mediterranean salad. Set ade and ade and ade and ade and

Open the pita pockets to serve. Spread a little amount of tahini sauce or Tzatziki sauce on a plate, then top with roasted chicken, arugula, Mediterranean salad, and pickles or olives, if desired. Serve monthondo

Chapter Six

EASY GREEN JUICE RECIPE

INGREDIENTS FOR ANY GREEN LENTIL SOUP RECIPE

Extra vrgn olve oil (Early Harvet) 1 large onion, chopped 2 carrots, 3 tablespoons dry oregano 1 tsp rosemary 1 12 teaspoon cumin

2 dry bay leaves 12 teaspoons red pepper flake

1 can mashed tomatoes 2 cups red lentils, washed and drained 7 cups low-odium vegetable broth alt koher

2 lemons, zest and juice

Garnish with fresh parsley

Optional: crumbled feta cheese INSTRUCTIONS

Hmmer but not moke 3 tablespoon extra vrgn olve ol onon, carrot, and garlic should all be added at this point. Cook for 3 to 4 minutes, turning every 3 to 4 minutes. Pce and bay leave should be included. Prepare a little amount of food for a few people.

econd tll fragrant, keep stirrng to keep pce fragrant frant

Crumbled tomatoes, broth, and lentil are all good additions. Seasoning with koher salt Bring to a boil, then reduce to a low heat for 15 to 20 minutes, or until the lentils are thoroughly cooked.

remove yourself from the heat Allow it cool somewhat before using a mmeron blender to purée if you have the time. Pulse a few times until you get the desired creamy consistency.

Return the soup to a high heat setting and stir to reheat it all the way through. Combine the lemon zest, lemon juice, and fresh parsley.

Fill a serving bowl halfway with the mixture and drizzle with extra virgin olive oil. Top each bowl with a liberal smear of fat cheese, if desired. SERVE wth your favorite cruty brew!

every almon UP INSTRUCTIONS

Extra virgin olive oil (I used Private Reserve Greek EVOO) 4 green onon, chopped 12 green bELL pepper, chopped 4 garlic cloves, minced 1 oz fresh dll, divided, chopped

1 pound fresh potatoes, carefully cut into rounds (best done with a mandoline slicer) 1 carrot, thinly cut into rounds (best done with a mandolin slicer)

1 tbsp. dried oregano 34 tbsp. coriander powder

12 teaspoon ground cumin

Kohr alt and black pepper lb salmon fillet, no kn, cut into big slices INSTRUCTIONS 1 lemon's zest and juice

In a big saucepan, heat 2 tablespoons extra virgin olive oil until it hums but does not smoke. Cook over medium heat, stirring often until fragrant (about 3 minutes). 12 to 15 to 20 to 30 to 40 to 50 to 100

Add the broth, potatoes, and carrots at this point. Season with kosher salt and black pepper before serving.

Bring to a rolling boil, then reduce to medium heat and cook for 5–6 minutes, or until potatoes and carrots are cooked.

Season with kosher salt and generously add to the pot of mmerging. Lower the heat and simmer for a few minutes until the salmon is cooked through, around 3 to 5 minutes, or until the almonds are cooked and flaky.

Stir in the remaining dill, lemon zest, and lemon juice.

Fill a serving bowl halfway with salmon. Serve with a serving of your favorite crunchy bread. Enjoy!

Falafel\sINGREDIENTS

DO NOT USE CANNED OR COOKED CHICKPEA.

12 tbsp oda

34 cup fresh cilantro leaves, stems removed 1 cup fresh parsley leaves

12 CUPS FRESH DILL, REMOVED 1 SMALL ONION, uartered

7-8 peeled garlic cloves To taste salt

1 tblsp ground black pepper 1 tblsp ground cumin 1 tblsp ground cinnamon 1 tblsp ground corander 1 tblsp ground cayenne pepper, optional tbsp roasted sesame seeds 1 tbsp baking powder Falafel Sauce ol for frying

Tahn Sauce FXING (OPTIONAL) for falafel andwch English cucumbers, chopped or diced, stuffed into pta pockets hopped or diced tomatoeS

INSTRUCTIONS FOR ARUGULA BABY PICKLES

(A day ahead of time) Place the drained chickpeas and baking soda in a large bowl with enough water to cover the chickpeas by at least two inches. Soak for 18 hours (or more if the chickpeas are still firm) over night. Drain the chickpeas well and set them aside to dry when ready.

To the large bowl of a food proceor ftted with a blade, add the chickpeas, herbs, onions, garlic, and spices. Run the food processor for 40 seconds at a time, or until everything is fully blended and a falafel mixture is formed.

Fill a container halfway with falafel mixture and close it securely. Refrigerate for at least 1 hour (or up to one whole night) before cooking.

Add the baking powder and egg yolk to the flaxseed mixture just before serving, and stir with a spoon.

Scoop tablespoons of falafel mixture into patty pans (12 inch in diameter). When forming the patties, it helps to have damp hands.

Fill a medium saucepan with oil until it reaches 3 inches above the surface. Heat the oil on high until it starts to bubble. Drop the flaxseed patties carefully into the oil and fry for 3 to 5 minutes, or until crispy and medium browned on the exterior. If required, falafel should be fried in batche to avoid crowding in the aucepan.

Drain the falafel patties in a condenser or on a plate lined with paper towels.

Serve hot falafel with other small plates; or arrange falafel patties in a pita bread with tahini or hummus, arugula, tomato, and cucumbers. Enjoy!

INGREDIENTS FOR EASY Roasted Tomato Basil Soup

lb 2–3 carrots, peeled and cut into tiny parts, roma tomatoes

Extra virgin olive oil (I used PRIVATE ReSERVE GREENS EVOO) ppper and salt

5 garlc cloves minced 2 medum yellow onons

2 ounces fresh basil leaves to 4 fresh thyme sprigs 1 cup canned crumbled tomatoes 2 tblsp. thyme 1 teaspoon oregano (dried)

paprika, 12 teaspoon

12 tsp. ground cinnamon 2 tbsp. water

OPTIONAL INSTRUCTIONS: SPLASH OF LIME JUICE

Preheat the oven to 450°F.

Combine the tomatoes and carrots in a large mixing dish. Season with kosher salt and black pepper after a generous drizzle of extra virgin olive oil. To combine, toss.

Transfer to a layer bakng heet and distribute evenly. Cook for around 30 minutes in a hot oven. Remove from the heat when ready and set aside to cool for 10 minutes.

Transfer the roasted potatoes and carrots to a large bowl fitted with a blade in a food processor. Blend with a little amount of water.

2 tblsp extra virgin olive oil, heated over medium-high heat until shimmering but not smoking in a large cooking pot Cook for about 3 minutes, then add the garlic and continue to cook until golden.

Into the cooking pot, pour the roasted tomato mixture. Crumbled tomatoes, 2 12 cup water, bal, thyme, and a pinch of salt and pepper are mixed together in a bowl. Add a pinch of kosher salt and black pepper to taste. Bring to a boil, then reduce to a low heat setting and partially cover. Let mmer for about 20 mnte or or or or or or or or or or or or or or or or

Remove the thyme stalks and transfer the tomato bal to a serving bowl. Add a dash of lime juice and a generous drizzle of extra virgin olive oil if desired.

Serve with crusty toast or grilled French baguette slices. Enjoy!

Greek-Style INGREDIENTS FOR BLACK EYED Pea Recpe I used Early Harvest Extra Virgin Olive Oil. Greek EVOO 1 big yellow onion, cut garlic cloves, chopped green bell pepper, peeled and chopped 3 carrots, peeled and sliced

12 teaspoon ground cumin 2 cup water 1 dry bay leaf 12 teaspoon paprika 1 teaspoon dried oregano

12 teaspoon red pepper flake, optional 15-ounce cans black-eyed peas, drained and rinsed 1 lime or lemon, juice of 1 cup fresh parsley INSTRUCTIONS

Heat extra virgin olive oil over medium heat, until it shimmers but isn't smoking, in a large pot or Dutch oven. onon, as well as garlic, should be added at this point. tranlucent and fragrant tranlucent and fragrant tranlucent and fragrant tranlucent and fragrant tr Add the carrots and bell peppers. Cook for 5 minutes, tossing every 5 minutes.

Add diced tomatoes (with their juices), water, bay leaf, pce, salt, and pepper at this point. Bring the water to a boil by increasing the heat. Incorporate the black-eyed pea. Bol for 5 mntere, then heat lower. Allow to boil for 25 to 30 minutes, partially covered (sometimes check to stir). Add a smidgeon of water if the black-eyed pea tew seems to be dry.)

Last but not least, tr in lemon juce and parley.

tranfer to bowls to erve. Drizzle some extra virgin olive oil on top. Serve with warm Greek pita or on top of orzo, rice, or your favorite grain.

INGREDIENTS: YUC

12 lb knle almon fllet, chopped

Djon mutard teapoon

2-3 tablespoon green onions, minced 1 cup freshly chopped parsley

1 teapoon ground corandER 1 teapoon ground UMAC

12 teaspoon paprika

12 tsp black pepper salt kosher

1 lemon 1 cup or ol

Burger Toppings with Salmon

Tztzk Sauce (recipe here) 6 oz baby arugula (more to your liking) 1 lced red onion

in order to serve

I frequently use whole wheat buns or Italian ciabatta rolls as an alternative to whole wheat buns. INSTRUCTIONS

Place 14 of the almon in the bowl of a large food processor. Add a lot of it. Run the processor until the mixture is ready. Place in a mixing bowl.

Place the remaining almon in the food processor and pulse a few times until coarsely chopped into 14-nch pieces (do not overprocess this second batch of almon, it should not get too fine or patty, it should t). Transfer to the same bowl as before.

Now add the minced green onion, parsley, and pce (corner, umac, paprika, black pepper). Season with kosher salt. Mx well until the mxture has been combined. Cover and chill for 12 hours.

Prepare the topping while the salmon is cooking. Tzatzk (Greek tzatzk) Succes according to the recipe. Prepare the arugula, sliced tomatoes, and remaining toppings and buns to serve.

Remove the almond mixture from the fridge when it is ready. 4 e ual parts dvd Form thnk patte of 1-inch thickness.

On a plate, place bread crumb. Place each pastry on the breadcrumb plate and coat one side, then flip over and coat the other side. Place the breaded almon patties on a parchment-lined sheet pan.

Preheat the oven to 350 degrees Fahrenheit and prepare the hamburger patties. 3 tablePOON EXTRA VIRGIN OLIVE Lower each of the patties with care and cook for 2 to 4 minutes, turning once, until lightly browned on both sides and medium-rare inside), (adjust heat as needed during cooking to keep things sizzling and cooking well without scorching the breadcrumbs.) (On an instant-read thermometer, the minimum internal temperature for medum-rare should be 115 to 120°F.)

Place cooked salmon burgers on paper towels to absorb any excess oil; season with Koher salt if desired. On top, squeeze in a squeeze of fresh lemon juice.

In a prepared bun, amble. Using a bit of tztzk sauce, spread the buns. Toss in the almonds, then top with arugula, tomato, and a single Ice... enjoy!

INGREDIENTS

I used Hojblanca for the xtra vrgn olve ol EVOO Spanh 1 large yellow onion, finely chopped 1 large garlic clove, chopped kosher salt and black pepper

12 teaspoon coriander, grated 12 tsp cumin powder

12 teapoON UMACE

12 tsp. red peppers, crushed 2 teapoON mint flakes, dried 1 tablespoon flour 6 cups low-odum vegetable broth 3 cups water, more if needed 12 ounces frozen cut leaf pnach, no need to thaw

12 cups green lentl or small brown lentl, rinsed 1 lime, juice of cups chopped flat leaf parsley INSTRUCTIONS

2 tablepoon olve oil, heated in a large ceramic or cast iron pot Cook until golden brown, then add the chopped onion. In a large mixing bowl, combine the garlic, all of the spices, the dried mint, the sugar, and the flour. Cook for 2 minutes on medium heat, stirring occasionally.

Add the blood and water at this point. Raise the heat to high and bring the liquid to a rolling boil; stir in the frozen potato and the lentil. Cook on high heat for 5 minutes, then reduce to medium-low heat. Cover and cook for 20 minutes or until the lentils are fully cooked. (Check the liquid level halfway through cooking and add a splash of hot water if necessary.)

Stir in the lime juice and chopped parsley after the lentils are fully cooked. Remove from heat and set aside for 5 minutes or so, covered. Serve hot with pita bread or a rustic Italian bread.

INGREDIENTS FOR ANY GREENSIDE EGGPLANT RECIPE

1.5 pound eggplant, cubed Kohler extra virgin olive oil (I used Private Reserve Greek EVOO) 1 large yellow onion, chopped 1 green bell pepper, tem and nnards removed, diced 1 carrot, chopped 6 large garlic cloves, minced 2 dried bay leaves 1 to 1 12 teaspoon sweet paprika or paprika that's been smoked 1 tblsp. organc corander

1 tbsp oregano (dried)

12 tp organc ground turmeric 34 tp grand cinnamon

12 tablespoons black pepper 28-ounce can of chopped tomato

Reserve the canning l ud for a 15-oz can checkpea. Herb uch a parley and mnt INSTRUCTIONS

Preheat the oven to 400°F.

Sprinkle salt over the eggplant cubes in a colander set over a big bowl or directly over your nk. Allow eggplant to "sweat out" any btterne by sitting on it for 20 minutes or more. Rinse and pat dry with water.

14 cup extra virgin olive oil, heated over medium-high heat until shimmering but not browning in a large braiser One, peppers, and chopped carrots are added. Cook for 2-3 minutes, stirring occasionally, before adding the garlic, bay leaf, pepper, and a dash of salt. Cook for a further minute, stirring constantly, until the mixture is aromatic.

Add in the eggplant, chopped tomato, chickpeas, and reheated chickpea lud now. To combine, stret

For about 10 minutes, bring to a rolling bol. Frequently stir Remove the top of the stove, cover it, and turn it on.

Cook for 45 minutes in the oven, or until the eggplant is fully cooked. (Check once or again while the eggplant is braising to see if any more liquid is required.) If that's the case, take it out of the oven for a few moments and slowly pour in 12 cup of water.)

Remove the eggplant from the oven and sprinkle with a generous amount of private sauce. Serve with fresh herbs (parsley or mint) as a garnish. Serve hot or cold with a serving of Greek yogurt or even Tztzk sauce and pta bread.

INGREDIENTS: Mediterranean Tuna Salad with Djong

Dreng for Zety Djon Mutard

2 12 teapoon good Djon mutard 1 lme zest

12 juice limes Early Extra vrgn olve harvet

12 teaspoon sumac, a pinch of salt, and a pinch of pepper 12 teaspoon crushed red pepper flake, optional When it comes to tuna, 3 can tuna, 5 ounce apiece (use high-quality tuna) 2 12 celery stalks, chopped 12 English cucumber, chopped 4-5 radishes, stems removed, chopped 3 green onions, white and green parts, chopped 12 medium red onion, finely chopped 12 cup ptted Kalamata olve, halved bunch parley, tem removed, chopped (about 1 cup chopped fresh parsley)

10-15 fresh mint leaves, stems removed, finely chopped (about 12 cup fresh mint chopped)

Optional Homemade Pta chp or pita pocket for serving, six slices heirloom tomatoes for serving, optional INSTRUCTIONS

In a small bowl, mix together the Djon mutard, lime zest, and lime juice to make the zesty mustard vinaigrette. Stir in the olive oil, sumac, salt, and pepper, as well as the crushed pepper flake (if using), until well combined. Remove yourself from the situation for a short time.

To create the tuna salad, combine the tuna, chopped vegetables, Kalamata olives, fresh parsley, and mint leaves in a large salad bowl. With a wooden spoon, mix carefully.

Dress the tuna salad with the dressing. Mx the tuna salad once more to ensure that it is evenly coated with the dressing. Before serving, cover and refrigerate for a half-hour. To the alad gently to refresh when ready to serve.

Serve in pta pockets for a dnner with a twist. Transfer to a serving platter and garnish with pta chup and laced heirloom tomatoes to serve as an appetizer. Serve a portion of the tuna salad on top of the licked heirloom tomatoes, if desired. Enjoy!

INGREDIENTS FOR MOROCCAN VEGAN TAGNE RECIPE

14 cup PRIVATE ReSERVE EXTRA vrgn olve ol, more for a later date

medium yellow onon, peeled and chopped 8-10 garlc clove, peeled and chopped 2 large carrot, peeled and chopped 2 large ruet potatoe, pe 12 tsp ground turmerc cup canned whole peeled tomatoeS 1 tbp Harissa pce blend 1 tp ground coriander 1 tp ground cinnamon 12 cup heaping chopped dred apricot

1 uart low-ODUM vegetable broth (or other vegetable broth) 1 lemon, juce of 2 cup COOKED CHICKPEAS

Fresh parley leaves in a handful INSTRUCTIONS

Heat olive oil over medium heat in a large heavy saucepan or Dutch oven until it is just hmmering. Increase the heat to medum-hgh and add one more. 5 minutes, tong regularly, saute

Add the garlic and all of the chopped vegetables. Salt & pepper to taste. t Cook, stirring often with a wooden spoon, for 5 to 7 minutes over medium-high heat. Tomatoes, apricots, and broth should be added at this point. Sean with jut a dah of alt again.

Cook for 10 minutes with the heat set to medium-high. Reduce the heat, cover, and cook for another 20 to 25 minutes, or until the vegetables have softened.

Cook for another 5 minutes on low heat, stirring occasionally.

Fresh parley and lemon juice Taste and adjust the seasoning, if necessary, by adding additional salt or harissa spice blend.

Switch to serving bowls and drizzle a good amount of cheese on top of each one. Private Extra virgin olive oil should be served on the side. Serve hot with your favorite bread, cucumber, or rice. Enjoy! Grains and Pata

INGREDIENTS FOR

Chapter Seven

SIMPLE MEDITERRANEAN OIL PATA

12 cup Early Harvet Greek Extra Vrgn Olive Ol (or Private Reserve Extra Vrgn Olive Ol) 1 pound thin paghetti

4 garlc cloveS, cruhed

3 scallions (green onions), top trmmed, both white and green chopped 1 teaspoon black pepper 6 ounces marinated artichoke heart, drained 14 cup puffed olives, halved 14 cup crumbled feta cheese, 10-15 fresh basil leaves torn

1 lemon (zested)

Optional: cruhed red pepper flaks INSTRUCTIONS

Cook the spaghetti pasta until al dente according to package directions (mine took 6 minutes to cook in plenty of boiling water with salt and olive oil).

Heat the extra virgin olive oil in a big cat ron kllet over medium heat when the pasta is almost done. Reduce the heat and add a pinch of salt and garlc. Cook, stirring often for 10 seconds. Toss in the parsley, tomatoes, and scallions that have been chopped. Cook for 30 seconds or so over low heat until barely warmed through.

Remove the pata from the heat, drain the cooking water, and return it to the cooking pot when it is ready. To Toss in the black pepper and re-cook.

To one more tme, combine the remaining components. Serve immediately in pasta bowls, garnished with more basil leaves and feta cheese if desired. Enjoy!

INGREDIENTS FOR Mediterranean roated vegetable barley r-ece

1 red bell pepper, cored, diced 1 medum red onon, diced salt and pepper tp/ 3.9 g harissa pce, dvded Harvest trmmed and chopped (both whte and green) greek extra virgin olve ol 2 callon (green onon) 2 oz / 56 g chopped fresh parsley 1 garlic clove, minced

2 tbsp/30 ml lemon juce (fresh squeezed) Taste with feta cheese (optional).

To taste (optional) roasted pine nut INSTRUCTIONS

Preheat the oven to 425 degrees Fahrenheit (230 degrees Celsius).

In a sauce pan, combine pearl barley and 12 cup water. Bring to a boil, then reduce to a low heat setting. Cover and cook anywhere from 30 to 45 minutes, or until the barley is cooked through (hould be tender but maintain a little chew.)

Put diced vegetables (zucchini, bell peppers, and red onion) on a large baking sheet while the barley is cooking. Season with salt, pepper, 12 teapoon smoked paprika, and 12 teapoon hara pce. Drizzle with a little more vrgn olve ol. To coat, to coat, to coat, to coat, to coat, to coat, to coat, to coat On the baking sheet, spread one layer evenly. Cook for 25 minutes or so in a preheated oven.

Remove any excess water when the barley is ready. Salt, pepper, 12 teaspoon harissa powder, and 14 teaspoon smoked paprika t

In a large mixing dish, transfer the cooked barley. Vegetables that have been roasted should be added. Chop the cauliflower, garlic, and parsley. Drizzle with lemon juice and extra virgin olive oil from the Early Harvest. Toss. Top with crumbled feta cheese and toasted pine nuts, if desired.

Serve hot, cold, or at room temperature! Enjoy.

Couscous\s

INGREDIENTS

1 cup low-sodium broth vrgn olive oil additional

Kosher 1 cup dry couscous ntant I utlized this coucouOptional to Flavor

a pinch of cumin (or any other spice)

1–2 garlic cloves, minced and cooked in extra virgin olive oil 2 general one, chopped

To your lkng, fresh plants INSTRUCTIONS: I used parsley and dill

Add broth or water to a sauce pan. A pinch of kosher salt and a drizzle of extra virgin olive oil To make a bol, combine all of the ingredients in a blender and process until smooth.

toat the coucou now. Heat around 1 to 2 tablespoons extra virgin olive oil in a non-stick skillet or pan. Add the cucumbers and stir with a wooden spoon until they are golden brown. This is an optional step that gives a delicious nutty flavor.

Stroucuu in the boled liquid as soon as possible. and turn off the heat immediately. Cover and let aside for 10 minutes, or until the cucumber has absorbed all of the broth or water.

With a fork, uncover and fluff.

You may eat the courgette simply or season it with spices and herbs for a more flavorful dish. Add a pinch of cinnamon, aged green onion, chopped green onion, and fresh herbs, if desired. Enjoy!

INGREDIENTS

34 pound spaghetti (or your choice of pasta) (I use Damond Crystal) Koher alt

Extra virgin olive oil (I use Privilege Reserve Greek extra virgin olive oil) 12 cup frozen peas 2 5- oz can solid albcore tuna, draned Zet of 1 lemon Juce of 12 lemon, more to your liking

1 oz. freshly chopped parsley 1 tablespoon drizzled oregano black pepper, to taste

6–8 ptted kalmata olved 1 jalapeno pepper (optional), grated To your long

INSTRUCTIONS

3 quarts water, 1 table poon koher alt, , 3 quarts water, Cook the pasta in boiling water until al dente (usually spaghetti takes 9 to 11 minutes to cook). After the pata has been cooking for 5 minutes, add the frozen peas and continue to cook with the pata for the remainder of the time. Take 34 cup of the cooking water and set it aside once the pata is ready. Preheat the oven to 350°F and drizzle the spaghetti into a casserole.

2 tablespoon extra vrgn olive oil, heated over medium-high heat until shimmering but not smoking in a large, deep cooking pan Cook, stirring occasionally, for 3 to 4 minutes with the red bell peppers. Cook, stirring constantly, for 30 seconds or until aromatic.

To mix, add the cooked pasta and peas to the pan. Add the tuna, lemon zest, lemon juice, parsley, oregano, black pepper, kalamata olives, jalapeño if using, and a generous sprinkling of Parmesan cheese. Drizzle in some extra virgin olive oil and some pasta cooking water as needed. Everything should be given a go. Taste and adjust the lkng to your preferences.

Into serving dishes, transfer the tuna pata. Enjoy!

INGREDIENTS FOR MUSHROOM BARLEY UP

Extra vrgn olve ol (I used Private Reserve Greek EVOO)

16 oz. baby bella muhrooms, well cleaned and halved or licked

1 yellon, chopped 4 garlic cloves, chopped 2 celery stalks, chopped 1 carrot, chopped 8 ounces white mushrooms, washed and cut 12 cup canned crushed tomatoes pepper, black

1 tblsp coriander 12 tblsp smoked paprika 34 tblsp

12 tsp low-odum broth (vegetable broth or beef broth) (12 tsp low- 12 cup packed chopped parsley 1 cup pearl barley rned

INSTRUCTIONS

Heat extra virgin olive oil over medium-high heat in a large Dutch oven until it shimmers but does not smoke. Cook for about 5 minutes or until the young bell mushrooms have softened and developed some color. Remove the contents of the saucepan and set it aside for the time being.

Add a smidgeon of extra virgin olive oil to the same pot. onon, garlc, celery, carrots, and chopped white muhroom Cook over medium-high heat for 4 to 5 minutes. Salt & pepper to taste.

Add the crushed tomatoes and spices (cumin, coriander, and smoked paprika). Cook for about 3 minutes, tossing occasionally.

Barley and broth Bring to a boil for 5 minutes, then reduce heat. Cover and cook for approximately 30 minutes over low heat, or until the barley is soft and fully cooked.

Back in the saucepan, add the cooked bella mushrooms and stir to combine. Cook for 5 minutes or so, or until the muhrooms are well warmed.

fnh wth recent parley Switch to ervng bowls and have a great time!

INGREDIENTS FOR A Medterranean COUCOU ALAD

Vnagrette Lemon-Dll

1 large lemon, plus a cup of extra virgin olive oil (I used Greek Private Reserve). 1 teaspoon dill, minced salt and pepper, 2 garlic cloves

Pearl Coucou for the Pearl

Couscous de Pearl PrIVATE ReSERVE EXTRA VIRGIN OLIVE Water

12 English cucumber, finely chopped 15 oz can chickpeas, drained and rinsed 14 oz can artichoke heart, coarsely chopped if required 3 oz. fresh mozzarella (or mozzarella cheese), optional INSTRUCTIONS

Place the vnagrette ngredent in a bowl and make the lemon-dll vnagrette. To combine, work together. Remove yourself from the situation for a short time.

Heat two tablespoons olive oil in a medium-sized heavy pot. Sauté the courgettes in the olive oil till golden brown. Cook according to package directions, using 3 cups boiling water (or the quantity specified on the container). Pour into a colander when ready. To cool, place the ade in a bowl.

Combine the remaining ingredients (excluding the bal and mozzarella) in a large mixing bowl. Then stir in the couscous and basil until everything is well combined.

Give the lemon-dill vinaigrette a good whirl and toss it in with the Coucou Salad. Mx a second time to combine. tet and adjut salt if necessary

Finally, mx mozzarella cheese. Garnh with a lot Enjoy!

INGREDIENTS FOR SIMPLE ITALY MINESTRONE SOUP

14 cup extra virgin olive oil (see our olive oil options here) 1 mall yellow onion chopped

2 carrotS

2 celery talk dced 4 garlc clove mnced 1 zucchini or yellow onion dced

1 cup fresh or frozen green beans, trmmed and cut into 1-inch pieces if required a pinch of salt and a sprinkling of black

paprika, 1 teapoon

12 tsp rosemary

6 cups vegetable broth or chicken broth 1 15-ounce can crushed tomatoes 15-ounce can kidney beans, grated parmesan cheese, and optional bay leaf (to 3 springs) handful of chopped par Fresh bal leaves in a handful

Serve with grated Parmesan cheese (optional)

marked

INSTRUCTIONS

Heat the extra virgin olive oil over medium heat in a large Dutch oven until it shimmers but does not smoke. Combine the onions, carrots, and celery in a large mixing bowl. Raise the heat to medium-high if necessary, and cook, stirring occasionally, until the vegetables are tender (about 5 minutes). Cook for a further minute, stirring often.

Combine the zucchini, yellow squash, and green beans in a large mixing bowl. Season to taste with paprika, rosemary, and a generous sprinkling of kosher salt and pepper. To mix the ingredients, toss them together in a bowl.

Add the mashed potatoes, broth, fresh thyme, bay leaf, and parmesan rnd now (if using.) Bring to a boil, then lower to a low heat and cover the saucepan completely. Allow for a 20-minute simmering time.

Add the kidney beans after uncovering the pot. Wait 5 to 10 minutes longer.

Finally, garnish with fresh basil and parsley. And, if ervng right away, trn the cooked pasta and mmer ever only to warm the pasta through; do not overcook. (For further information, see Cook's Tip #2.)

Remove the bay leaf and the cheese rind. Taste and adjust the lighting to your liking. Serve hot minestrone in dinner dishes with a sprinkling of grated Parmesan cheese (optional).

NOTES

Note: The pata is already cooked before being added to the mixture; merely follow the package directions. You'll begin with one cup of dry pasta, which will yield two cups of cooked pasta.

Cook's Tip #1 (Create It Yourself): Minestrone is designed to be customized, so use any vegetables and beans you have on hand to create your own recipe. It's common to add a handful of pnach or diced potatoes. Instead of kidney bean, you may use wheat bean or a mixture of both. Feel free to omit the potatoes if you're looking for a low-carb option. Add cooked ground turkey or even leftover rotisserie chicken if you want something more substantial. Cook's Tip #2 (Make--Ahead): Once the onion is cooked, add the carrots and celery. If you are not serving the minestrone right away, wait until you are ready to add the cooked pasta to the pot. This will give you the best results and prevent the pasta from absorbing too much broth and becoming too soggy.

TIP #3 for Meal PREPURATION: Keep the cooked pasta out if you want to make mnetrone for lunch over multiple days. Simply add a small amount of the pasta to your bowl, followed by an appropriate amount of hot magnesium.

Baked Cod Recpe wth Lemon and Garlc

INGREDIENTS

a pound 14 cup chopped fresh parsley leaves, 4-6 pieces Lemon Sauce is a sauce made with lemons.

5 tblsp freshly squeezed lemon juice 5 tblsp extra vrgn olve ol

2 tblepoon melted backet 5 crushed garlic cloves

Cooking

1 tblsp flour (all-purpose)

1 tblsp coriander, ground 34 tblsp sugar 12 teaspoon black pepper paprika, 34 teaspoon ground cumin, 34 teaspoon tea powder,

INSTRUCTIONS

Preheat the oven to 400 degrees Fahrenheit (200 degrees Celsius).

In a hallow bowl, combine the lemon juice, olive oil, and melted butter (but not the garlic). Set ade and ade and ade and ade and

Combine all-purpose flour, powdered sugar, salt, and pepper in a small bowl. Place yourself next to the lemon juice.

Remove the fish from the water and set it aside to dry. Dip the fish in the lemon sauce before dipping it into the flour mixture. Excess flour should be shaken away. Keep the lemon sauce refrigerated until you're ready to use it.

Warm 2 tablepoon olve ol in a cast-iron skillet (or an oven-safe pan) over medium-high heat (watch the ol to make sure it is shimmering but not smoking). Add the fh and ear to each side to add color but don't completely cook (approximately 2 minutes each side). Turn off the heat in the skillet.

Add the grated garlic to the remaining lemon sauce and mix well. Drizzle over the fillets in a circular motion.

Bake in a preheated oven until the fh flakes easily with a fork (10 minutes should enough, but start checking sooner). Remove from the heat and top with parsley. Immediately serve.

one pan medterranean baked halibut recept wth vegetable

INGREDIENTS

Sauce:

2 lemons, 2 lemon juice, 2 lemons, 2 lemons, 2 lemons, 2 lemons, two lemons, two lemons, two lemons, two lemons, two lemons, two lemons, two lemons 1 12 tbp greek extra vrgn olive ol 1 tbp greek dll weed 1 tbp seasoned salt, more for later 12 tp ground black pepper 1 tp dried oregano 12 to 34% teapoon greek dll weed

fh

1 pound fresh green beans 1 lb cherry tomatoes 1 big yellow onion halved

12 pound halibut filet, cut into 12 inch pieces INSTRUCTIONS

Preheat the oven to 425 degrees Fahrenheit (230 degrees Celsius).

Whisk together the auce ingrediants in a large mixing bowl. Toss in the green beans, tomatoes, and onions with the sauce to coat. Transfer the vegetables to a large baking sheet (21 x 15 x 1 inch baking sheet, for example) using a big slotted spoon or spatula. Keep the vegetables to one side or half of the baking sheet, and make sure they're all spread out in one layer.

Add the remaining sauce to the halibut fillets and toss to coat. Place the halbut fillet on top of the vegetables on a baking sheet.

Lightly prnkle the halibut and vegetable wth a lot more eaoned alt.

Cook for 15 minutes at 425°F in a preheated oven. Then, tranfer the bakng heet to the top oven rack and brol for another 3 mnute or so, watching carefully. The chrysanthemum tomatoes hould begin to pOP up and

Remove the baked halibut and vegetables from the oven when they are ready. Serve with a side of your favorite grain, Lebanese rice, or pata. A robust salad, such as this Mediterranean Three Bean Salad, is an excellent addition.

INGREDIENTS FOR Moroccan FISH

(I used Private Reserve EVOO) Extra Virgin Olve Ol 8 garlic cloves, divided (4 minced garlic cloves and 4 minced garlic cloves) 1 15-ounce can chickpeas, drained and rinsed 2 tablespoons tomato paste, medium tomatoes, diced 1 red pepper, chopped, lced 1 and a half gallon (1.2 gallons) of water

1 cup fresh cilantro black pepper and kohr alt

12 pound fish fillet piece (about 12 nch in thickness) 1 12 tp Ra El Hanout

paprika (34 tblsp)

12 tblsp lemon juice

INSTRUCTIONS

Heat 2 tablespoon extra vrgn olve ol (I used Private Reserve) in a big pan with a cover over medium heat until it shimmers but does not smoke.

Cook for a few minutes, stirring often, until aromatic. Combine the tomato paste, diced tomato, and bell peppers in a mixing bowl. Cook, stirring often, for 3 to 4 minutes over medium heat.

Add the chickpeas, water, cilantro, and cut green onions now. Salt and pepper to taste.

12 tsp Ras El Hanout powder mixture If necessary, raise the heat and bring the mixture to a boil. Reduce the temperature of your home. Cover and cook for about 20 minutes with the lid part-way. (Check periodically and, if necessary, add a little water.)

In a small mixing bowl, combine the remaining Ra El Hanout with the cinnamon and the paprika. Season both sides of the fish with kosher salt and pepper, as well as the spice combination. A generou sprinkle of extra vrgn olve Work the spices and olive oil into the fish to ensure that it is evenly covered.

When ready, add the seasonings to the pan and nestle the chicken pieces into the saucy chickpea and tomato mixture. Drizzle a little sauce over the top of the fh. Cook for 10 to 15 minutes more over medium-low heat, until the fish is fully cooked and flaky. More fresh clantro garnh.

Serve with your favorite crunchy bread, grain, or rice right away.

INGREDIENTS

lb knle chcken breat (boneless) pepper and salt

2 tsp oregano (dried) 1 tsp. thyme 1 tsp. thyme Paprika (Sweet) 4 grallic cloves, minced 3 tblsp vrgn olve olve olve olve olve olve olve ol 12 lemon juice 1 medium red onion, quartered and thinly sliced 5 to 6 Campari tomatoes, or small Roma tomatoes, quartered and thinly sliced For garnh, a handful of freshly picked parsley

INSTRUCTIONS FOR FRESH BASIL LEAVES FOR GRAIN

Preheat the oven to 425 degrees Fahrenheit (200 degrees Celsius).

Drizzle some dry on the chicken. Set a cooked chicken breast in a big zip-top bag and zip the top (making sure to let any air out first), then place it on your poultry cutting board. With the use of a meat mallet lke the one, flattened the checken Rep with the rest of the fried chicken pieces.

Season the chicken on both sides with kosher salt and pepper, then transfer to a large mixing basin or dish. Spices, grated garlic, extra virgin olive oil, and lemon juice are added to the pan. Combine to ensure that the chicken is completely covered with pce and garlic.

pread the onon slices on the bottom of a large lightly oiled baking dish or pan. Place the seasoned chicken on top and finish with the tomatoes.

Cover the baking dish completely with foil and bake for 10 minutes covered, then uncover and bake for a further 8 to 10 minutes or so. Carefully observe. Depending on the thickness of your chicken breasts, this may take less or more time. Use an instant digital cooking thermometer to make sure the chicken is fully cooked. The temperature should be 165 degrees Fahrenheit.

Relocate yourself away from the heat. Allow 5 to 10 minutes for the chicken breasts to rest before serving (cover with foil or another pan). Remove the cover and top with fresh parsley and bal. Enjoy!

INGREDIENTS

1 14 lb large shrimp or prawns, peeled and deveined (thaw first if frozen) 1 tblsp flour (all-purpose)

1 to 2 teapoon more

12 tsp. pepper and 12 tsp. salt

12 teaspoon ground cinnamon 14 teaspoon cayenne 14 teaspoon sugar tablepoon butter Ghee clarified butter is what I like. Extra virgin olve oil, 3 tablePOON

12 red onion, thinly sliced 4 garlic cloves, chopped 12 green bell pepper and 12 yellow bell pepper, cored and chopped 2 tablespoon dry white wine tablepoon fresh lemon juice 1 cup canned diced tomato 1 cup chicken or vegetarian broth

INSTRUCTIONS FOR

Chapter Eight

CUPPED PARSLEY

Place the shrimp in a wide bowl and let them dry. Combine the flour, smoked paprika, salt and pepper, curry powder, cayenne pepper, and sugar in a large mixing bowl. Until the hrmp is well covered.

Melt the butter with the olive oil over medium heat in a large cast iron kettle. Garlc and hallot Cook for 2-3 minutes, stirring occasionally, until fragrant (be careful not to burn the garlic). Cook for another 4 minutes or so, stirring occasionally, before adding the bell peppers.

Add the hrmp next. Cook for 1–2 minutes before adding the chopped tomatoes, broth, white wine, and lime juice. Cook for a few minutes more or until the hrmp develops a brilliant orange color.

Finally, tr nto the chopped fresh parley and erve!

INGREDIENTS

Salmon should be prepared as follows:

Koher alt Extra virgin olve ol (I used Early Harvet Greek extra virgin olve ol) lb almon fillet

12 lemons, cut into round parsley

To make a lemon-garlic sauce, combine the following ingredients in a small mixing bowl.

1 large lemon, juice of 2 lemons, 1 tablespoon extra virgin olive oil (I used Early Harvest Greek extra virgin olive oil) 2 tp dried oregano 5 garlc cloves, chopped 12 teaspoons black pepper 1 teaspoon weet paprka INSTRUCTIONS

Preheat the oven to 375 degrees Fahrenheit (190 degrees Celsius).

Create the lemon-garlc auce. Mix the lemon juice, lemon zest, extra virgin olive oil, garlic, oregano, paprika, and black pepper together in a small bowl or measuring cup. Giving the sauce a good whirl is a good idea.

Prepare a heet pan lined with a big piece of fol (large enough to drape over the almoon). Apply eXTRA vrgn olive ol on the foil's top.

Now, pat the almoon dry and season with kosher salt on both sides. Place it on the flanned heetpan. Top with lemon garlic sauce (be careful to evenly distribute the sauce).

Cover the almon with foil (seam side up). Bake for 15 to 20 minutes, or until salmon is almost entirely cooked through at the thickest portion (cooking time may vary depending on thickness of fish). If your almon is thicker, check it a few minutes early to make sure it doesn't overcook. It may take a little longer if your piece is really thick, 12 inches or more.)

Remove the almon carefully from the oven and open the foil to reveal the top. Place in the broiler for 3 minutes or so, depending on how crispy you want it. Keep a close eye on it as it broils to ensure it doesn't overcook or burn.)

INGREDIENTS

2 medium zucchini, 11 oz., halved lengthwise, then half moons
1 red pepper, cored and cut into chunks

1 red onion, handled

9 oz. baby broccoli trmmed and cut into bite-size pieces 12 lb. boneless chicken breast

Koher salt and black pepper, minced 5 garlic cloves 2 to

1 tblsp. prka

1 teaspoon coriander powder

1 zetted and squeezed lemon white vinegar, 1 teaspoon

I used some extra vrgn olve ol Greek PRIVATE RESOURCE EVOO Optional fresh parley for garnh

INSTRUCTIONS

Preheat the oven to 400 degrees Fahrenheit (200 degrees Celsius).

In a large mixing basin, mix the sliced vegetables. mnced garlc and chcken peces Seasoning made from kosher salt and black pepper. pce is a word that should be added to your vocabulary. Now stir in the lemon zest, lemon juice, vegetables, and a generous drizzle of extra virgin olive oil. Toss everything together well, ensuring that the vegetables and chicken pieces are uniformly coated.

In a large sheet pan, transfer the cooked and vegetables. In one layer, spread nicely.

Bake for about 20 minutes in a preheated oven until the chicken is well cooked. Place under the brighter brefly if you'd want additional color.

Before serving, garnish with fresh parsley (optional).

INGREDIENTS FOR MEDIEVAL SALMON KABOB

a pound Approximately cut samon fillet into cubes 1 ncm – 12 ncm or n size 1 zucchini, sliced into rounds 1 tiny onion, sliced into rings For marinade, koher salt and pepper

14 cup extra virgin olive oil (I used Early Harvest Greek olive oil) to cup extra virgin olive oil 1 lemon, zested and juiced 3 garlic cloves, minced 2 tablespoons chopped fresh thyme leaves 2

tablespoons dried oregano 1 tablespoon ground cinnamon (I used the Aleppo pepper)

12 tbsp coriander, grated INSTRUCTIONS

In a small bowl, combine the marinade ingredients of extra virgin olive oil, lemon juice, and zest, garlic, oregano, thyme, cumin, Aleppo pepper, and coriander in a small bowl.

In a large mixing dish, combine almon pie, zucchini, and onions. Season to taste with kosher salt and pepper, and mix vigorously. Pour the marinade over the almon once more, making sure it's fully coated. Allow for 15 to 20 minutes of marinating time.

Starting with the almond, thread the almond, zucchini, and onion through the kewer (if using wooden kewers, make sure they've been soaked for 30 minutes before using).

Preheat an outside grill (note: ndoor grilling note). Cover the grill with salmon kewers. Grill the salmon skewers for 6 to 8 minutes, covered, or until the flesh is opaque throughout, turning once halfway through cooking (the easiest method to flip the salmon skewers is using tongs).

INGREDIENTS: Sauted Shrimp and Zucchini in a Mediterranean Style INGREDIENTS: Sauted Shrimp and Zucchini in a Mediterranean Style INGREDIENTS: Sauted Shrimp and Zucchini in a Mediterranean Style INGREDIENTS: Sauted Shri

12 teaspoon ground corander 12 teaspoon sweet paprika lb large shrimp prawns, peeled, and deveined tablepoon Extra vrgn olive ol I used Private Reserve Greek EVOO

12 finely sliced medium red onion minced and divided 5 garlic cloves

1 bell pepper corrected and laced into sticks

1–2 zucchini, lengthwise, licked into 12 moons (you may use 1 zucchini and 1 yell uah)

12 cup cherry tomatoes, halved 1 cup cooked chickpeas from canned chickpeas

kosher pnch alt black pepper in a pinch

lemon juce of 1 large

Fresh bal leaves, torn or cut into ribbons (you may use any herb according on what you have on hand)

INSTRUCTIONS

Combine the pce (oregano, cumin, cinnamon, and paprika) in a small mixing bowl.

Place the shrimp on a dry plate and season with kosher salt and 12 tsp of the spice mixture. Set aside for a short time or save for later. (Save the rest of the pce mxture for the veggies.)

Heat 2 tablespoons extra virgin olive oil over medium heat in a large cast-iron pan. Cook for 3 to 4 minutes, until aromatic (do not let the garlic burn).

Zucchini, bell peppers, and chickpeas are all good additions. Season with salt and pepper, as well as the rest of the spice mixture. t t t a t a t a t Raise the heat a little and cook the vegetables until soft, stirring occasionally (about 5 to 7 minutes).

For the time being, transfer the vegetables to a big plate. Return the kllet to the heat and add a lttle btt Add the remaining garlic and the seasoned hrmp. Cook, stirring occasionally, over medium-high heat until the shrimp is completely cooked (approximately 4 to 5 minutes).

Back into the kllet with the hrmp, add the cooked veggies. Combine the cherry tomatoes and lemon juice in a large mixing bowl. Give everything your best shot. Finish with a pinch of fresh basil.

Baked fish with tomatoes and capers in a Mediterranean style

INGREDIENTS

cup Private Reserve 1 small red onion, finely chopped large tomatoes, diced (3 cups diced tomatoes) Greek extra virgin olive oil If you want, use quality canned tomatoes.)

ten garlc cloves, chopped

12 tblsp. organic ground conditioner

1 tblsp. weet 1 teaspoon cumin powder (organic)

cayenne pepper (12 tsp) (optional) capers (12 tbsp)

seasonings golden rank

1 12 pound white fish fillet (wild if possible) such as cod fillet or halibut fillet 12 lemon juice (or more)

1 lemon's zest

To garnish, use fresh parsley or mint.

INSTRUCTIONS

Prepare the tomato sauce and the caper aioli. Heat extra virgin olive oil in a medium saucepan over medium-high heat until it begins to shimmer but does not smoke. Cook for 3 minutes, or until it begins to turn a golden color, tossing occasionally. Toss in the tomatoes, cheese, pepper, and a pinch of salt (but not too much), as well as the pepper, capers, and ran. Bring to a boil, then reduce to medium-low heat and leave to simmer for about 15 minutes.

Preheat the oven to 400°F.

Fh deer and eaon wth alt and pepper on both deers.

Fill the bottom of a 9 12" x 13" baking dish with 12 of the cooked tomato sauce. Arrange the fh atop the table. Toss in the lime juice and zest, then finish with the remaining tomato sauce.

Bake for 15 to 18 minutes in a 400°F preheated oven, or until flaky (do not overcook). Remove from heat and garnish with fresh parsley or mnt, depending on your preference.

Serve hot with grilled zucchini from the Middle East, Greek potatoes, or Lebanese rice.

Chapter Nine

CONCLUSION

Though there is no one-size-fits-all Mediterranean diet, this dietary trend is generally high in healthy plant foods and low in animal foods, with a focus on fish and seafood.

It's been linked to a slew of health benefits, including the ability to control blood sugar levels, promote heart health, and improve cognitive function, among others.

The best part is that you can adapt the Mediterranean diet's principles to suit your needs. If you despise almonds and sardines but enjoy whole wheat pasta and olive oil, start by creating a delectable Mediterranean-inspired meal with your favorite ingredients.

CPSIA information can be obtained
at www.ICGtesting.com
Printed in the USA
LVHW020805060422
715456LV00007B/272

9 781804 385937